FOODS THAT HEAL OSTEOPOROSIS

ANN MARIE LUCAS

DISCLAIMER

For legal reasons, we are obliged to say the following.
The publishers have carefully checked the contents of this
book to ensure that it is as accurate as possible at the time
of publication.
This book is for information only. Please be advised that the
information on these pages does not necessarily represent
the views of health professionals and physicians. Do not
treat this as a substitute for medical advice from qualified
doctors.
If you are pregnant, we advise you to seek professional
advice before making any dietary changes. In the case of
any emergency, such as an accident, high fever, or heart
attack, please seek medical attention immediately. If you
are worried that you may have a severe illness, please
consult a medical professional before following any tips in
this book.

FOREWORD

Are you tired of feeling like osteoporosis controls your life? Are you seeking a comprehensive, holistic approach to healing your body naturally? Look no further. *Foods That Heal Osteoporosis* is your guide to reclaiming control over your bone health and revitalizing your life.

In this persuasive and insightful guide, you will embark on a transformative journey to understand, address, and conquer osteoporosis through holistic methods. From unraveling the mysteries of osteoporosis to exploring the critical role of calcium in bone health, each chapter equips you with essential knowledge and practical strategies to embark on your healing journey.

Discover the bewildering truths about Calcium supplements and learn how to optimize calcium absorption for maximum effectiveness. Dive into a world of healing foods and unlock the power of nutrition in combating osteoporosis. Indulge in mouthwatering recipes designed to nourish your bones and invigorate your body.

However, healing is not just about what you put into your body but also about how you move it. Explore targeted physical exercises tailored to strengthen your bones and improve your overall well-being, empowering you to live life to the fullest.

Do not let osteoporosis dictate your life any longer. Take charge of your health, embrace holistic healing, and embark on a journey towards a more substantial, healthier you. Your body deserves nothing less.

This guide will tell you all about:

- The best form of calcium: which one is the best?
- The medical findings about drugs for Osteoporosis
- Is calcium alone enough for healing osteoporosis?
- Are calcium supplements good enough?
- What kind of milk products work?
- What are the key recipes?
- Fourteen recipes to inspire you

Here is what you can expect in this guide:

In Chapters 1 and 2, there is a quick understanding of what happens to your body when osteoporosis occurs and then an understanding of calcium and how it works. Finally, what kinds of calcium are optimum for your body?

Chapters 3 and 4 cover the biological systems involved in healing osteoporosis and the foods that nurture them.

Chapter 5 is a valuable collection of recipes that will contribute to the well-being of the circulatory, digestive, and skeletal systems and help heal osteoporosis.

Chapter 6 is a set of simple exercises that will help bone mass.

So, if you want to better results, read on:

However, promise yourself that you will do what it takes to get a life of comfort and mobility.

CHAPTER I

HOW OSTEOPOROSIS OCCURS

The Skeleton Lives!

Our bones are alive! They are continuously being renewed: old bone is removed, removed, and replaced with new bone.

We continue to build bone until our early thirties, and then our bodies work to retain existing bone.

OSTEOPOROSIS DEFINED

Osteoporosis is a condition characterized by a decrease in the density of bone, weakening in strength, and resulting in fragile bones.

Bones become weaker or "porous" when old bone is removed faster than new bone is rebuilt. As a result, bones become brittle and break or fracture easily in osteoporosis.

This disorder of the skeleton weakens the bone and results in frequent fractures (breaks) in the bones. The most common being fractures of the spine, hip, and wrist.

Bones affected by osteoporosis can break with relatively minor injury that usually would not cause bone fracture. The fracture can be either in the form of cracking (as in a hip fracture) or collapsing (as in a compression fracture of the vertebrae of the spine). The spine, hips, ribs, and wrists are common bone fractures from osteoporosis, although osteoporosis-related fractures can occur in almost any skeletal bone.

In the light of these bone-breaking nightmares, read on and help yourself towards having solid bones and towards easing pain and curing yourself.

OSTEOPENIA: A LESSER FORM OF THE DISEASE

Osteopenia is a condition of bone slightly less dense than normal bone but not to the degree of "porous" bone in osteoporosis.

OSTEOPOROSIS EXPLAINED

This is due to a process called **bone resorption.** This is the process by which osteoclasts (a type of bone cell that removes bone tissue) break down bone and release the minerals, resulting in a transfer of calcium from bone fluid to the blood.

This results in porous bones.

Abnormally porous bone is compressible, like a sponge.

The Cause of Osteoporosis

Calcium is leached from the bones because there is insufficient calcium for the body to function.

If there were enough calcium in the body, there would be no need to leach the calcium in the bones.

The skeleton serves as a resource bank for calcium. When there is insufficient calcium in the body, it can borrow calcium from the skeleton. When enough calcium is taken by the individual, this borrowed calcium is returned to the skeletal system.

However, when the individual does not intake enough calcium, the calcium that has been borrowed is not returned to the skeleton. The bones then have "holes, " making them less stable, much weaker, and easier to break.

Why Calcium is so Important

In males, there are about 3 pounds or about 1.4 kg of calcium, and in females, about 2 pounds or 1 kg of calcium. Calcium is the most abundant mineral in our bodies.

99% of calcium is found in our bones and teeth and the other 1% in soft tissues and watery body parts.

The Function of Calcium in Our Bodies

(Sourer, 1995; Whitney et al., 1996; Sizer et al., 1997)

- Calcium is responsible for constructing, forming, and maintaining bones and teeth.
- Calcium is a vital component in blood clotting systems and helps heal wounds.
- Calcium helps to control blood pressure, nerve transmission, and release of neurotransmitters (chemicals used for signaling in the brain).

- Calcium is essential in producing enzymes and hormones that regulate digestion, energy, and fat metabolism.
- Calcium helps to transport ions (electrically charged particles) across the membrane.
- Calcium is essential for muscle contraction.
- Calcium assists in maintaining all cells and connective tissues in the body.
- Calcium may help reduce the incidence of premature heart disease, especially if adequate magnesium intake is also maintained.
- Calcium may help to prevent periodontal disease (gum disease).

The Effects of Calcium Deficiency

(Sourer, 1995, McCarron et al, 1987; McCarron et al, 1991)
Calcium Deficiency, in conjunction with high sodium intake, is related to a higher risk of hypertension.
Calcium Deficiency can lead to calcium loss from the bone (initially from the jaw and the backbone), which can lead to deformity.
Calcium Deficiency can cause extreme nerve sensitivity, muscle spasms, and leg cramps (called tetany) at deficient blood levels.

Osteoporosis Lurks

Herein lies our problem. Suppose 1% of calcium is not supplied daily for our body to function normally. In that case, it will leach on the calcium in the bones and keep taking it from them until osteoporosis occurs.

The worst part is that while this process is occurring, most of us are unaware of it. Many people are already suffering from osteoporosis or osteopenia but are not aware of it until they have pain.

But most people do not know of it until they have a fracture.

There may be no signs or warnings.

Women are in the danger zone because of pregnancy, lactation, and menopause and are told to look out for it by public health systems.

Osteoporosis can mean the difference between living healthily and losing your independence and mobility in old age. One in four people who experience a hip fracture requires skilled care for at least a year after the injury. In older adults, a hip fracture later in life increases the chance of death by up to 20%.

The Flipside of Calcium

High doses (several grams) of calcium may cause blood calcium levels to rise and lead to calcium deposits in soft tissue, such as the heart and kidney (Somer, 1995).
Large calcium intakes may reduce zinc and iron absorption and impair vitamin K metabolism (Somer, 1995; Gregor, 1988).
Very high blood levels of calcium can cause heart or lung failure.
Calcium ascorbate or calcium citrate are safe. They are less toxic than calcium from oyster shells (Whiting, 1994).
Calcium from oyster shells may have lead levels that exceed the amount considered safe for children.

Calcium Deficiency in Females - Postmenopausal:

From the RDA table, you will see that menopausal women need calcium the most. This is because osteoblasts, the bone-building cells, contain progesterone receptors, and this hormone encourages bone-building. (Please note that bone building is done at age 30, but bone, as in all cells, needs to be renewed and replaced.) After menopause, progesterone, a female hormone, is deficient, so bone formation is also lacking.

Progesterone works with estrogen to conserve calcium within the body and limit the withdrawal of calcium from the bones. After menopause, this relationship does not exist.

Calcium: RDAs (Recommended Daily Allowance)

Infants aged 0-05 need 400 mg
Infants aged 0.5-1 need 600 mg
Children from 1-10 years need 800 mg
Males and females from 11-24 years need 1200 mg
Males and females from 25-50 years need 800 mg
Pregnant and lactating women need 1200 mg
Post-menopausal females on estrogen therapy need 1000
Post-menopausal females NOT on estrogen therapy need 1500
Post-menopausal females over the age of 65 need 1000

The Challenge of Calcium Intake

So, how much calcium should we take? And if we supplement it, will it be taken directly into the bloodstream in exactly the amounts we would like?

Normal bone comprises protein, collagen, and calcium, all strengthening bone.

Calcium is absorbed into the system only if magnesium, zinc, fluoride, and phosphorous work together.

This means that if you were to take the RDA of calcium into your system without other minerals such as magnesium, zinc, fluoride, and phosphorous, it would not be absorbed by the small intestine.

The amount of phosphorous, calcium, and calcium to magnesium is essential in these minerals' absorption, use, and excretion.

Do not forget that high calcium levels in the blood can cause a blockage of arteries and can cause heart or lung failure.

What is the Medical Answer to Osteoporosis?

The medical treatment of osteoporosis involves the prevention of osteoporosis rather than therapy per se.

It recommends:

Lifestyle changes, including quitting cigarette smoking, curtailing excessive alcohol intake, exercising regularly, and consuming a balanced diet with adequate calcium and vitamin D
Medications that stop bone loss and increase bone strength have side effects. Many drugs that are used to treat osteoporosis are widely known as **Bisphosphonates.**

How Bisphosphonates Work

"They are FDA approved and of an essential natural bone-building chemical, pyrophosphate, which normally helps bind calcium to bone tissue through a process known as mineralization. Unlike pyrophosphate, however, bisphosphonates *block normal mineralization and osteoclastic bone resorption.*

"In normal bone remodeling, osteoclasts first resorb bone tissue, forming little pits in the bone structure. In short order, osteoblasts come along—like microscopic road repair crews—to fill those pits with healthy new bone. Under normal circumstances, osteoblasts remain inactive until the osteoclasts first do their thing. If osteoclastic activity is suppressed enough, though, as it is by bisphosphonates, osteoblasts have no cavities to fill, so the formation of new bone ceases. Although estrogens also inhibit osteoclastic activity, they do so naturally and do not suppress osteoblastic bone building, which agents like progesterone, testosterone, or strontium can still stimulate.

Thus, the physical cost of bisphosphonate-induced bone stabilization is to freeze normal bone remodeling—a highly unnatural state of affairs."

-from Dr Lane Lenard, PhD

Bisphosphonates aim to stop bone fractures- but instead, it increases the chances of some fractures.
These drugs increase the risk of 'atypical' fractures – these are fractures to the femoral bone, which extends from the hip to the knee.
The doctors also ask you to drink more milk, but studies

have shown that the more dairy we consume, the more bone we lose.

It also showed that the more we consumed yogurt, cheese, and other dairy products, the more we were at risk of fractures.

This is because dairy products have about ten times more calcium than magnesium. Magnesium is essential to calcium absorption.

My advice is that you do not need to avoid milk, but you may need to take it in moderation... only when you feel like it. Try not to make it a daily routine!

The only way to seriously heal osteoporosis is through intelligent food intake.

One thing remains clear: Osteoporosis is mainly a lifestyle disease. There is good evidence that exercise and diet alone can prevent it.

Osteoporosis is linked to our modern, protein-rich diets. We eat up to five times the protein our bodies need, and the acid byproducts of protein leach calcium and other minerals from our bones.

More calcium is needed when dietary protein, fat, or phosphorous is in excess.

Many people mistakenly believe osteoporosis occurs simply due to a calcium deficiency. In reality, many factors play a part in bone building and subsequent bone loss. Along with calcium, our bodies require adequate boron, copper, magnesium, manganese, silica, and zinc. Folic acid, vitamin B_{12}, and vitamin D are essential as well.

What You Have Learnt So Far in Chapter 1... A Recap

Our bones are continuously being renewed. Old bone is

being replaced by new bone every day. Moreover, if this is the case, then we have healthy bones.

Osteoporosis results from calcium being leached from the bones because of insufficient blood supply.

A lack of calcium in the blood supply implies you are not eating calcium-rich food.

Osteopenia can be the onset of calcium deficiency. While more than 70 million worldwide suffer from osteoporosis, there are many millions more who have osteopenia and are not aware of it. Are you one of them?

Calcium is essential because 99% of calcium is found in the bones and teeth.

Calcium helps digestion, blood clotting, muscle contraction, enzyme production, and maintenance of cells and connective tissues. It also reduces premature heart disease and prevents gum disease.

Calcium deficiency is related to hypertension, bone loss, skeletal deformity, extreme nerve sensitivity, muscle spasms, and leg cramps.

An over-supply of calcium in the system can lead to calcium deposits in the heart and kidney, upset vitamin K and iron absorption, and even cause lung failure.

1 in 3 women over 50 suffer from osteoporosis.

The RDA of calcium for males and females over 50 is about 1200 and 1500mg, respectively.

Calcium alone will not be the answer to a solution for osteoporosis.

The medical answer to osteoporosis is bisphosphonates. They block normal mineralization. It is a halfway measure that ceases the formation of new bone.

The only way to seriously heal osteoporosis is through intelligent food intake.

CHAPTER 2

BEWILDERING TRUTHS ABOUT CALCIUM SUPPLEMENTS

Facts about Calcium You Need to Know

Osteoporosis is debilitating. The pains that come with this ailment are severe (if and when they do arrive). Medical science does not have a cure. It only recommends ingesting more calcium in the form of supplements and bisphosphonates.

Medical science says that enough calcium will make bones healthy again. However, our bodies need enough calcium; instead, they excrete too much of what they already have. The balance lies in what type of calcium is easily absorbed by your body and how it does that.

Read on and find out.

Is calcium only necessary for the bones?

No. While 99% of calcium is in the bone, the 1% in the blood is crucial for vascular contraction, vasodilation, muscle function, nerve transmission, intracellular signaling, and hormonal secretion. So, this 1% is vital for metabolic functions. Too much calcium in the blood can lead to cardiovascular and kidney issues.

If you do not have enough calcium in your diet, your body will take it from your bones to ensure normal cell function, which can lead to osteoporosis. Calcium deficiency can contribute to mood problems such as irritability, anxiety, depression, and difficulty sleeping.

A study (2010) that involved 12000 women taking calcium supplements (of about 1000mg a day) showed that there was a 27% increased risk of heart attacks.

So, the question is, do you have enough calcium in your system? If so, how do you know? Moreover, if not, how do you know?

Here is one way to find out...

How Much Calcium Do You Have?

You could go for a Bone Mineral Density (BMD) test:

Optimal BMD is between a +1 and a -1

Osteopenia = 1.0 to 2.5

Osteoporosis = lower than 2.5

You would have to go to a doctor for your yearly check-up and ask for the BMD test.

Taking Calcium Supplements Alone Is Not Enough:

If you take calcium without magnesium, it will not be absorbed into your body. It will be excreted.

It would be best to take calcium with adequate amounts of vitamin D to be accepted by your body.

Calcium without zinc in your system is not going to work

Calcium without manganese is ineffective

Calcium without copper, too, is not going to work either

Calcium Supplements: Carbonate or Citrate?

There are two primary forms of calcium: calcium carbonate and calcium citrate.

You should take the carbonate - the more common form - if your digestive system is more acidic than alkaline. It requires extra stomach acid to be better absorbed. This is to be taken after meals.

If you have gas, bloating, constipation, or a combination of these symptoms and acid reflux, you know that your system tends to be more acidic than alkaline.

You should take the citrate if you want to take it at any time of the day, with or without food. It is the more easily absorbed form of calcium. It does not require extra stomach acid.

If you suffer from acid reflux, avoid calcium citrate. Calcium citrate has also been known to increase the absorption of aluminum from foods (Somer, 1995). If you are taking calcium citrate, avoid antacids with aluminum in them.

There is also dolomite, bone meal, or oyster shell. These are naturally occurring calcium but may contain heavy metals or lead. Avoid.

Calcium Gluconate and Calcium Lactate: You must take more in smaller doses of elemental calcium.

Coral calcium is composed of calcium carbonate. It makes too many claims that seem doubtful.

Look for Elemental Calcium on the Labels

While the bottle of your calcium supplement tablets may claim to give you 500mg of calcium carbonate, it will provide only 200 mg of elemental calcium.

This means it will provide just the 200 mg, not the 500 mg.

Look for Elemental calcium content. Elemental calcium is listed in the Supplement Facts Panel.

How Much Calcium Should You Take at a Time?

As already stated, the amount of calcium absorbed depends on the elemental calcium taken at one time.

The body can handle only 500mg at any one time.

So, if you need 1000mg of calcium daily, remember to split the dose. Take 500mg in the morning and the other 500mg in the evening.

Calcium Excretion by the Body

If you take more than the required amount of calcium in the body, then it should be eliminated. Sometimes, with supplement intake or milk intake, this is not possible.

When we eat unhealthily, calcium gets eliminated as well.

If you take high amounts of sodium and protein, this would increase calcium excretion.

High intakes of caffeine can also increase calcium excretion and reduce absorption.

Alcohol intake can reduce calcium absorption

Carbonated soft drinks can reduce calcium absorption

Calcium is Useless Without....

Calcium is absorbed within your system and works well only in combination with

Magnesium

Phosphorous

These trace minerals

Zinc,

Fluoride,

Boron

Copper

Iron

Manganese

And these vitamins

Vitamin D

Vitamin K

Vitamin C

All these must be taken in the correct ratios.

Cal-Mag: The Best of Friends

Without magnesium, nothing will be absorbed within your system if you take calcium alone.

However, with magnesium, calcium can stick around and help your bones. The ideal ratio is two parts calcium to 1 part magnesium.

So, for 1000 mg of calcium, you would need about 500 mg of magnesium.

The Recommended Daily Amount for magnesium is 400 mg. (do keep in mind that absorption rates are not high, so taking a higher amount than the RDA is not a problem)

The body can store calcium well, but magnesium is quickly eliminated, so it is rare to have an excess of magnesium in your system. Magnesium is vital for healthy bones as it regulates calcium absorption into the bones.

- Calcium stimulates the nerves, while magnesium works to calm them.

- Calcium helps form blood clots, while magnesium promotes blood flow to prevent excessive clotting, which, as you understand, will lead to atherosclerosis.

The Problem with Dairy

Dairy products have about ten times more calcium than magnesium. This causes a problem for the system. Calcium can damage the system when there is insufficient magnesium to act positively on the bones. It can clog arteries and cause heart problems.

The more dairy we consume, the more bone we lose. Despite all the **calcium** dairy contains, some believe its high protein content can cause osteoporosis. When protein is digested, it increases the blood's acidity. The body then pulls **calcium** from the blood to neutralize the acid.

As calcium is an alkaline mineral, the body is thought to sacrifice calcium from the bones to neutralize the rise in blood acidity. However, calcium from the bones is then excreted in the urine and not recycled, leaving a calcium deficiency.

Milk also contains D-galactose, a type of sugar. Experimental evidence in animals has suggested that D-galactose is associated with aging and damage to tissues at a cellular level. Researchers say an injected dose of 100mg/kg of D-galactose has been shown to accelerate biological signs of aging in mice, equivalent to 6 to 10g in humans, or the amount found in one to two glasses of milk.

One large-scale Harvard research followed 72,000 women for two decades and found no evidence that drinking milk could prevent bone fractures or osteoporosis. Another study of more than 96,000 people found that the more dairy men consumed as teenagers, the more bone fractures they experienced as adults. Similarly, another study found that teenage girls who consumed the most calcium, mainly in the form of dairy products, were at greater risk for stress fractures than those consuming less calcium.

How Much of Vitamin D is Needed?

Vitamin D increases calcium, magnesium, and phosphorous absorption.

The recommended dietary intake is 400.

However, this depends on the climate you are living in. If you have long winters, you should up the intake.

The best way to get vitamin D is to stay in the sun. If you are fair-skinned and stay in the sun for about 20 minutes daily, you will get your share of Vitamin D.

If you are darker skinned and have more melanin, stay in the sun for about 30 minutes daily and get your fair share of Vitamin D.

That leads to the following essential partner of calcium...

The Relationship Between Phosphorous and Calcium

Phosphate makes up more than half the mass of bone mineral. (Do not confuse that with the fact that 99% of calcium is found in your bones!)

Bone health deteriorates when calcium and phosphorous are not balanced. When phosphorous is too high, calcium is leached out of the bones, which becomes brittle.

So, too much phosphorous is bad for the system, as is too little phosphorous.

When there is too little phosphorous in the system, it will not bind with any extra calcium supplement you take. Then, the calcium will not be absorbed in the system.

You need to have about 700g of phosphorous in the system.

If the diet is low in phosphate, more calcium supplements are needed.

Take a supplement that has both calcium and phosphorous in it.

Trace Minerals

The intake of **fluoride** required by the body is minimal, at 2.5 mg daily, but still necessary for the hardening and stabilizing of bones. There is no need to take individual supplements of fluoride.

Zinc, iron, manganese, and **copper** help our bodies to form the optimal bone matrix or structure for bone strength. Calcium supplementation may reduce the absorption of both zinc and copper. Zinc can also increase the rate of bone loss and the onset of osteoporosis.

The RDA for zinc is 11mg for boys and 8 mg for men and women.

The RDA for copper is 0.9mg

The RDA of iron is between 8-18 mg

The RDA for Manganese is 2.3 mg for men and 1.8 mg for women.

Boron may enhance the absorption of calcium and estrogen metabolism.

Vitamin C and Vitamin K

Both help in forming the bone matrix for bone strength.

Vitamin K, along with vitamin D, modulates bone mineralization. It positively affects calcium balance.

New studies show that vitamin C intake discouraged fracture risks. It showed a protective effect on the bone health of older adults.

Vitamin C can counter oxidative damage that would usually break down bone structure. It also helps in healing damaged bones.

What you have learned so far in Chapter 2... A recap

- Taking calcium supplements of 1000mg a day can lead to increased risks of heart attacks
- Take a BMD test to know whether you have osteoporosis or Osteopenia
- Calcium carbonate or calcium citrate? The best one depends on your diet. Although calcium carbonate seems safer, it has less absorption than calcium citrate. The absorption of calcium citrate may be up to 60%, and the carbonate up to 30%
- Read the amounts of elemental calcium on the labels of your calcium supplement bottle
- The body can handle only 500 mg of calcium at a time
- High intake of calcium can be dangerous to our health
- Even if we take calcium from natural foods, calcium can still be eliminated if protein intake is too high. This is also the same for too much caffeine intake, too many carbonated drinks, or even too much oxalic acid, as found in spinach
- Calcium cannot be absorbed without the correct ratios of magnesium and phosphorus
- Other trace minerals such as zinc, fluoride, boron, copper, iron, manganese, and vitamins D, K, and C are essential.

CHAPTER 3
THE BEST HEALING FOODS FOR YOUR BODY

Medical science has already admitted it: it has no absolute answer to heal osteoporosis completely.

The answer to healing Osteoporosis is the food you take into your body. This chapter will act as a guide to understanding the Healing Power of Natural Foods.

The story of healing foods is not simply one of resolving osteoporosis but also of life enrichment and well-being. Many people live at only 50% of their full health potential, not really sick but not truly well either. This is the plight of people living with osteoporosis. Suppose you start eating foods that heal by rebuilding your bones. In that case, these foods will enhance wellness by increasing the efficiency and energy levels of underactive endocrine glands and all other organs, including bones, muscles, nerves, joints, veins, and arteries.

If, like most human beings, you are doomed by your local physician to have been diagnosed with osteoporosis, and you accept that as a life-long fate with no resolutions to it, that is the whole battle lost!

However, you must be patient. This is a process that takes time to fix. The body needs time to balance all that's gone wrong. As read in the previous chapter, many minerals are out of balance in your body, leading to this dis-easeful condition you are in now. If you want ease to be present in your life again, give the foods time to heal. Give yourselves six months to a year, and all will be well. A minimum of 6 months!

So, the first thing to do is to frame your attitude positively: nobody has more power over your body's health than you have. It depends on what you choose to put in it. If your cupboard is untidy and disorganized, is it anyone's fault other than yours? Can you blame the housekeeper? (Particularly if you do not have one!) No, no, the onus is all yours and yours alone. Moreover, in cleaning it and making it work properly again, the onus is all yours and yours alone!

Hippocrates, the Father of Medicine, also believed in the importance of Natural Remedies, such as diet. Natural forces within us are the true healers of disease. Healing is a matter of time, but it is also a matter of opportunity. Everything in excess is opposed to nature.

Healing is a Matter of Time

If you have studied Chapter 2, you will note that the chemical processes in the body due to building bone strength are very complicated. It begins with the digestive system. Whether or not nutrients are well absorbed depends on the cleanliness of the digestive tract, particularly the small intestines. If the small intestine is clogged with "old dirt" and has not been appropriately cleared, then the small intestines' villi cannot absorb nutrients as efficiently. This may present a problem with the appropriate calcium, phosphorous, and magnesium levels absorbed in the body.

Hence, there may be a need to cleanse the bowels first.

Eating the correct foods just for osteoporosis alone will begin the cleansing of the bowels.

However, this WILL take time—up to six months.

The 12 Body Systems

The 12 body systems control the life process in the body. These systems are the following:

1. Skeletal

2. Muscular

3. Respiratory

4. Endocrine

5. Digestive

6. Reproductive

7. Integumentary/Skin,

8. Lymphatic,

9. Excretory

10. Circulatory,

11. Nervous

12. Urinary

Let us examine three systems: the skeletal, the digestive, and the circulatory systems.

Each of these systems has a function. Of course, each interacts with the other to maintain balance in the body. If there is a calcium deficiency supplied through the digestive system, the body will tap the skeletal system for calcium to compensate. Whatever neglect is shown in one system, another will compensate for it.

This law of equilibrium and balance can work positively, too. If we help one system to better itself, it will also benefit the other systems.

For example, if we eat correctly, the digestive and excretory systems will function smoothly. Nutrients are carried to the circulatory system and the endocrine system. In this way, many, if not all, systems are aided.

Foods for the Skeletal system

Structure	Function	Vitamins	Minerals	Foods	Drinks	Herbs
All bones and cartilage	Support protect body, leverage mineral storage, red blood cell production	C, D, A, B complex, B₁, B₁₂, B₆, Folic Acid, Niacin, Pantothenic Acid, Bioflavonoids	Fluorine, Calcium, Copper, Iodine, Zinc, Sulfur, Sodium, Silicon, Iron, Potassium, Phosphorous, Magnesium	Sesame seed, kale, millet, celery, barley, okra, almonds, collards, turnip greens, raw goat's milk, Black figs	raw goat's milk, black cherry juice, green kale juice, celery/parsley juice, veal joint broth	Comfrey, kale, chicory, juniper berries, arnica flower, elderflower, oat straw, alfalfa, Irish moss

Foods for the skeletal system *Structure:* All bones and cartilage

Function: Support and protect the body, leverage mineral storage, red blood cell production

25

Vitamins: C, D, A, B complex, B_2, B_6, B_{12}, E, Folic Acid, Niacin, Pantothenic Acid, Bioflavonoids

Minerals: Fluorine, Calcium, Copper, Iodine, Zinc, Sulfur, Sodium, Silicon, Iron, Potassium, Phosphorous, Magnesium

Foods: Sesame seed, kale, millet, celery, barley, okra, almonds collards, turnip greens, raw goat's milk

Drinks: raw goat's milk, black cherry juice, green kale juice, celery/parsley juice, veal joint broth

Herbs: Comfrey, kale, chicory, juniper berries, arnica flower, elderflower, oat straw, alfalfa, Irish moss

Foods for Digestive System

Structure	Function	Vitamins	Minerals	Foods	Drinks	Herbs
Gastro-intestinal tract with exception of large colon, salivary glands, liver, gall bladder, pancreas,	Mechanical and cellular breakdown of food for cellular use,	B_1, B_2, B_6, B_{12}, D, E, K, Folic Acid, Inositol, Niacin, Pantothenic Acid	Sodium, Chlorine, Magnesium, Potassium, Iron, Sulfur, Copper, Silicon, Zinc, Iodine	Papaya, liquid chlorophyll olives, swiss chard, celery, kale, beet greens, whey, shredded beet, watercress, yoghurt	Parsley juice, papayas juice, carrot juice, chlorophyll juice, potato peeling broth, whey drinks	Papaya, alfalfa, aloe vera, peppermint, slippery elm, cayenne, burdock, comfrey, ginger, fennel, anise

Foods for the skeletal system *Structure:* All bones and cartilage

27

Function: Support and protect the body, leverage mineral storage, red blood cell production

Vitamins: C, D, A, B complex, B_2, B_6, B_{12}, E, Folic Acid, Niacin, Pantothenic Acid, Bioflavonoids

Minerals: Fluorine, Calcium, Copper, Iodine, Zinc, Sulfur, Sodium, Silicon, Iron, Potassium, Phosphorous, Magnesium

Foods: Sesame seed, kale, millet, celery, barley, okra, almonds collards, turnip greens, raw goat's milk

Drinks: raw goat's milk, black cherry juice, green kale juice, celery/parsley juice, veal joint broth

Herbs: Comfrey, kale, chicory, juniper berries, arnica flower, elderflower, oat straw, alfalfa, Irish moss

Foods For The Circulatory System

Structure	Function	Vitamins	Minerals	Foods	Drinks	Herbs
Heart blood vessels blood	Distribute oxygen and nutrients, transport carbon dioxide and waste from cells; acid/base balance; regulate body temperature; form blood clots	B Complex, B_6, Niacin, C, E, Bioflavonoids, Choline, Folic Acid, Inositol	Calcium, Iron, Silicon, Cobalt, Magnesium, Iodine, Phosphorous, Zinc, Potassium, Manganese, Nitrogen, Sulfur, Fluorine	Brewer's yeast. garlic, wheat germ, liquid chlorophyll, alfalfa sprouts, buckwheat, sun dried olives, watercress, rice	Blackberry parsley juice, black fig juice, watercress parsley juice, grape juice, Hawthorne berry tea	Hawthorne berry, cayenne, ginger, garlic, burdock, echinacea, red clover, oat straw

Foods for the Circulatory system

Structure: Heart blood vessels blood,

Function: Distribute oxygen and nutrients to cells; transport carbon dioxide and waste from cells; acid/base balance; regulate body temperature; form blood clots

Vitamins: B Complex, B_6, Niacin, C, E, Bioflavonoids, Choline, Folic Acid, Inositol

Minerals: Calcium, Iron, Silicon, Cobalt, Magnesium, Iodine, Phosphorous, Zinc, Potassium, Manganese, Nitrogen, Sulfur Fluorine

Foods: Brewer's yeast. garlic, wheat germ, liquid chlorophyll, alfalfa sprouts, buckwheat, sun-dried olives, watercress, rice

Drinks: Blackberry/parsley juice, black fig juice, watercress/parsley juice, grape juice, Hawthorne berry tea

Herbs: Hawthorne berry, cayenne, ginger, garlic, burdock, echinacea, red clover, oat straw

If you look at all three systems, i.e., the skeletal, the digestive three systems, i.e., the skeletal, digestive, and circulatory systems, you would see that under the vitamins listing, they tend to coincide. So does the mineral column.

If you look at the food column, foods such as kale, liquid chlorophyll, alfalfa, celery, and watercress are repeated through the systems.

Here's the key: If you include kale, greens, alfalfa, celery, and parsley in your diet, you cannot go far wrong.

The variety of food and the various ways of cooking will give you your answers. If you cook these combinations always in the same way, you may not be able to help yourself stick to your nutritious diet for healthy bones.

Still, I would like to stress that no one magic bullet will make you better. Health exists through many good foods. Good sense and proper nutrition point the way to a state of wellness that safeguards against imbalance and disease.

Source: Jenson B, 1993, Foods that Heal, Avery publishing group, New York

What you have learned so far in Chapter 3... A recap

Medical science does not claim to have a cure for osteoporosis.

You must persevere, allow time to heal, and stay positive to heal yourself.

The body systems that you are concerned with are the skeletal, digestive, and circulatory and the foods associated with them

FOUR STEPS TOWARDS STRONG BONES

You can source calcium and the necessary balance of minerals for correct absorption into the intestinal walls in many foods.

This is why I set out the table for the digestive system: if the digestive system is clogged, whatever good food you take for osteoporosis will not be absorbed by your body's system. So, first things first.

Answer these questions:
Do your bowels move with ease every day?
Do you eat enough fiber (whole grains, fruits, vegetables?)
Do you drink enough water? About six glasses? (water means water...not teas, colas, and coffee.
Do you take wholegrain flour, brown bread, and raw (brown) sugar into your system daily?
If you answer yes to all 4 of those questions... yay! ... you have an excellent digestive and excretory system.
If you answer yes to 3 of those questions, that is still good.

If you answer yes to 2 or less, ... your digestive system is in trouble. Moreover, you need help with it.

Step 1: Towards clearing your digestive system

A regimen for cleansing your digestive system for one week (two weeks if you have the discipline)

1. Make sure to eat papaya
2. Drink aloe vera rigorously at least once a day
3. Include greens in your diet for a week,
4. Take the potato peelings broth twice a day for a week.
5. Avoid gluten and wheat products during this one week.
6. Try to include turmeric in your diet, e.g., yogurt with a pinch of turmeric.
7. Avoid red meats (in fact, try to go vegetarian for a week if you can)
8. Get enough fiber into your system: Eat fruits, nuts, and greens
9. Get eight glasses of water in a day.

That should clear the system quite quickly. Now, your digestive tract is ready to absorb all the vitamins, minerals, and particularly calcium you are prepared to feed it.

Step 2: Identify the food with the highest calcium levels:

Here is a list of foods that are the highest in calcium

Keep in mind that RDA for calcium per day is 1000mg.

*Cheese gruyere, 283 mg per 100 gm,

*Cheese parmesan, 1376 mg per 100 gm,

FOODS THAT HEAL OSTEOPOROSIS

*Cheese, most others, 212 mg per 100 gm,

*Skim milk, 125 mg per 100 gm,

*Whole milk, 113 mg per 100 gm,

Almonds, 226 mg per 100gm,

Brazil nuts, 160 mg per 100gm,

Broccoli, 80 mg per 100gm

Brussels sprouts, 78 mg per 100gm

Canned Sardines, 382 mg per 100 gm,

Carrots, 37 mg per 100 gm

Celery root, 37 mg per 100gm

Chicory, 71 mg per 100gm

Chilli powder, 278 mg per 100 gm,

Coconut milk, 41 mg per cup

Collard greens, 112 mg per 100gm,

Corn meal– I cup, 50 mg

Currant, 59 mg per 100gm

Dandelion greens, 188 mg per 100gm,

Dates, 63 mg per 100gm

Egg –medium-sized, 55 mg

Endive, 72 mg per 100gm

Figs, 54 mg per 100gm

Flax seeds, 225 mg per 100gm,

Garlic, 25 mg per 100 gm

Herring, 74 mg per 100 gm,

Kale, 147 mg per 100gm,

Lemon, 61 mg per 100gm

Lentils, 80 mg per 100gm

Lima Beans, 28 mg per 100 gm

Molasses, 205 mg per 100gm,

Mustard greens, 129 mg per 100gm,

Okra, 73 mg per 100gm

Onions, 25 mg per 100gm

Orange, 28 mg per 100gm

Parsley, 205 mg per 100gm,

Parsnip, 45 mg per 100 gm

Raspberry, 29 mg per 100 gm

Raw turnip greens, 190 mg per 100gm,

Rice – brown boiled, 20 mg per cup

Sesame seeds, 989 mg per 100gm,

Sweet potato, 26 mg per 100 gm

Tofu, 372 mg per 100gm,

Turnip, 33 mg per 100 gm

Watercress, 196 mg per 100gm,

Whey powder, 796 mg per 100 gm,

Whole wheat bread, 107 mg per 100 gm,

Yoghurt, 183 mg per 100 gm,

Note: *While milk products show a high calcium reading, they are not easily absorbed in the body. Much of the calcium is wasted.

Spinach is not listed here because of its very high oxalic acid content that negates the calcium in it.

Step 3: Identify Super Calcium foods

The five super calcium foods are:

1. Sesame seeds 989mg per 100 gm

2. Whey is a by-product of cheese making. It is used to produce ricotta. It is very high in calcium and a host of other minerals. If you can get hold of whey powder, make some drinks from them, or be inventive and sprinkle them over salads and use it in soups (to thicken them) and dishes.

You can use Sweet Whey Powder while baking. Sweet whey powder can replace 15% of flour in a recipe.

Use the Sweet Whey powder to give structure to your dough and batter. Almost 50% of the eggs used in cake recipes can be replaced with whey powder.

Sweet whey powder can be used in the 1-5% ratio per total volume of ingredients in the recipe of white bread, pizza dough, and cookies.

3. Tofu is very high in calcium. *One half-cup serving of tofu has 227 gm of calcium.*

4. Cheeses

5. Turmeric

Turmeric is the new food for osteoporosis.

A recent study has established that turmeric can prevent osteoporosis and bone loss.

Turmeric comes from a plant related to ginger. It has been used since time immemorial in India as Ayurvedic medicine. It has been used for many illnesses, injuries, wounds, coughs and colds, stomach aches, and arthritis.

How to use turmeric in your everyday cooking

It is widely available as a spice; you may buy it as pills or supplements. However, let me advise you to use it in your cooking as often as possible: when you stir-fry vegetables or grill any meat, try sprinkling some onto the food - for vegetables, about half a teaspoon, and for meat, about one teaspoon.

How turmeric works

Turmeric. Research at the University of Arizona by Jane Funk found that it prevented both arthritis and the development of bone loss that fosters bone resorption and bone destruction around the joint. It prevented the loss of bone mineral density and the spongy, porous bone found in the spine and the hip, the types of bones most subject to fracture.

Turmeric is a source of vitamins B6 and C and minerals like iron, potassium, magnesium, and manganese. Turmeric has antioxidants, of which curcumin is the most active.

Turmeric is anti-microbial, anti-bacterial, anti-ulcer, and works as an antiseptic and antibiotic. It is also an anti-inflammatory agent.

Step 4: Eat your way to healthy bones.

If you try to include these five foods daily, you are on your way to recovery. Use them in creative ways and every day. Some recipes have been included with these foods in mind. Please read the following chapter and try them out. They will help you with osteoporosis and are delicious.

A reminder: This is not a magic pill you only take once. It is a magic pill (provided by Nature) that you must take continuously for at least a year. (depending on how severe your condition is).

What You Have Learnt So Far in Chapter 4... A Recap

- Your digestive system: the importance of the absorption powers of intestinal villi
- Step 1: Clearing the digestive system: Eating the right foods for a great digestive system
- Step 2: List of foods highest in calcium
- Step 3: The five calcium superfoods
- Step 4: Eat your way to healthy bones

CHAPTER 5

RECIPES THAT HEAL OSTEOPOROSIS

The Secret

THE KEY RECIPE

Here is a recipe that could go a long way to improve your bone health. It is through natural foods. Moreover, because it is through natural foods, and your body knows how to balance itself, you need not worry about the ratio of calcium to phosphorous to magnesium and so forth… because they are all balanced well in these foods!

My suggestion is to include a spoonful of this mixture during breakfast: either on your toast or your cereal, and you would get your needed amounts of calcium, phosphorus, and magnesium +trace minerals all in one go…. Doesn't it sound like that magic pill?

10 almonds

10 walnuts

3 Brazil nuts

5 tablespoons of sesame seeds

5 tablespoons of oats

2 tablespoons of barley

5 tablespoons of bran

10 figs

4 prunes

You could sprinkle some of this over a salad too.

Method:

Coarsely grind the almonds, sesame seeds and oats.

Grind the 2 tablespoons of barley really fine.

Crush the walnuts and brazil nuts with the flat part of a large knife

Cut the figs and the prunes into tiny pieces.

Mix everything along with bran. Store in an airtight bottle in the refrigerator.

Notes for the recipe above:

Almond has oil and lecithin, which are brain, nerve, and gland foods. It also has magnesium manganese, phosphorous iron, zinc, copper, potassium, and selenium. It is the best of nuts to use.

Almonds are also a powerhouse of vitamin E, niacin, B1, B2 folate, B6, and pantothenic acid.

Sesame seeds are the highest and best source of calcium (half a cup has about 700mg of calcium), copper, magnesium, and zinc. They are the champion of all seeds. They have the perfect ratios for calcium absorption into our bloodstream. They also contain most of the vitamins necessary for bone strength.

Walnuts are a great source of omega-3 fatty acids and calcium. It is an excellent manganese, copper, magnesium phosphorous, zinc, iron, and selenium source. They also contain traces of iodine.

Walnuts contain vitamins B1, B2, B6, vitamin E, and niacin.

Brazil nuts contain strontium, a trace mineral crucial for increasing bone mineral density. Only 1-3 mg of it is needed daily.

Barley has iron, magnesium, phosphorous, calcium, potassium, sodium, selenium, fluoride, zinc, and copper.

It has vitamins B2, B6, niacin, folate, riboflavin, vitamin E, and vitamin K.

Oats have calcium, magnesium, phosphorous, potassium, zinc, vitamin B complex, iron, zinc, and manganese.

It has inositol, which is essential for maintaining blood cholesterol levels.

Bran is high in calcium, iron, magnesium, phosphorous, potassium, manganese, and selenium. It also has zinc and copper.

Bran also has vitamin B complex, vitamin E, Vitamin K, folate, pantothenic acid, and choline.

Figs are high in vitamin K, choline, calcium (245mg found in 600g), magnesium, potassium, and phosphorous. They also contain zinc, copper, selenium, and manganese.

Prunes are a good source of vitamin B and vitamin K (which is essential for bone strength)

It is high in calcium, magnesium, phosphorous, and potassium. It also has zinc, copper, manganese, fluoride, and iron.

*** This recipe contains calcium from various food sources, which is necessary for bone thriving. Be sure to take a generous spoonful with your breakfast every morning. Moreover, do not worry that it is not in the right proportions... with natural foods, the body knows what to do.

KEY SALAD

Try to have this salad every day. This salad is instrumental in giving you the right amounts of calcium. One lady I know personally healed herself of osteoporosis by taking this salad daily for lunch with rye bread. She avoided gluten and had one apple for dinner. She did stretch exercises regularly. She continued with this regime for two years before she was free of osteoporosis.

lettuce leaves

1 carrot, grated

1 beetroot, grated

1 tablespoon ginger, grated

1 lemon, juiced

1 orange cut into pieces

Sprinkle a tablespoon of sesame seeds over it

Note: Beetroot has minimal traces of calcium. It is a food with oxalates that can defy calcium absorption. However, research has indicated that this interference is relatively small, and it still allows calcium to penetrate the system, particularly if your digestive tract is healthy. Oxalates only really become a problem if you suffer from kidney stones.

Beets are a source of heart-healthy folate and potassium and are an excellent source of the antioxidant manganese. Beets are also a good source of digestive-supportive dietary fiber, vitamin C, and bone-healthy magnesium, copper, and iron.

CHERRY JELLY

Desserts with lunch or dinner: An excellent way to end your meal. Gelatin has lots of calcium in it. You do not need to add sugar if you make a cherry jelly. This is lovely food, especially for rheumatism and for strengthening your bones. Gelatin is what you have to use to build up your body when you get arthritis and osteoporosis.

1 package cherry cherry-flavored gelatin

3 cups boiling water

1 cup cold water

1cup ice cubes

1 can pitted dark sweet cherries

OR

1 cup cherry concentrate

Method

Combine cherry-flavored gelatin and 1 1/2 cups boiling water in a bowl; stir until gelatin dissolves (about 3 minutes).

Add 1 cup cold water and 1 cup ice cubes; stir until ice melts. (If using cherry concentrate, then add now. Skip steps 3 & 4. And chill)

Chill until the consistency of unbeaten egg white (about 10 to 15 minutes).

Fold in cherries.

Pour into a 13 x 9-inch baking dish. Cover and chill until set.

Note: Cherries are suitable for an elimination diet. It should not be mixed with dairy. It has a high alkaline content and helps get rid of toxic waste. It is a gall bladder and liver cleanser because of its high iron content.

It also has calcium, phosphorous, vitamin A thiamin, riboflavin, and niacin.

THE AYURVEDIC REMEDY FOR OSTEOPOROSIS

100g of white sesame seeds, hulled.

Brown rice boiled ½ cup

Method

1. Grind sesame until very fine in a dry grinder, and then add a small amount of sesame oil until you get a good paste.

2. Boil some brown rice

3. Eat the brown rice with the sesame paste

4. You may eat it with salad or stir-fried vegetables, too.

Note: **Sesame seeds are one of the foods highest in calcium. It has 989 mg of calcium per 100 grams**. Sesame seed butter can be purchased in health food stores in raw organic form. You may use this instead. Nevertheless, beware that these are only with hulled sesame seeds. The hulls of sesame seeds contain oxalic acid that nullifies calcium. This process happens in the digestive system.

Remember that you cannot get too much calcium from natural products...if the body notices a surplus, it will release it accordingly.

Rice is a good source of minerals; while a cup of boiled rice only has 20 mg of calcium, it has a lot of magnesium, phosphorous, copper, and manganese. All are necessary for bone health. It also has essential omega 3 and 6, a source of vitamin B and pantothenic acid.

BARLEY AND KALE SOUP

6 cups water

450 g potatoes, unpeeled and cut into quarters

230g kale, washed, stripped from their stems and finely shredded

4 tbsp barley

59 ml. extra virgin olive oil

1 large onion, peeled and cut into quarters

Freshly ground black pepper

Salt to taste

Method

Prepare the kale and put it aside.

Bring water to a boil; add potatoes, onions, and salt.

POTATO PEEL BROTH*

2 cups of potato peeling

2 cups celery,

1 cube of vegetable stock

2 cups of carrot tops

1 medium onion

1-liter water

Method

Finely chop all ingredients, add to water, boil, and simmer for 20 minutes.

Strain and drink one or two cups a day. Store for up to 2 days.

Note: This broth is high in organic sodium and potassium, which assist in restoring calcium balance.

*The above recipe is from B Jenson, 1908 **Dr Jensen's Book of Nutrition: A Daily Regimen for Healthy Living**. Keats Publishing, Chicago*

BARLEY, KALE, AND CHICKEN SOUP

(8 servings) you may want to halve the ingredients for a smaller serving

550ml carton chicken brot,h or if you do not have this, mix 500ml water with one chicken cube stock

1/2 bunch celery

1/2 bunch kale, cut up

2 teaspoons minced garlic

1 can tomatoes, undrained, diced

1/2 can tomato sauce

equal amounts of water to the desired consistency

3 cups mixed vegetables (fresh or frozen, carrots, celery root, broccoli, bok choy, zucchini)

1/2 cup pearl barley

1/2 cup peeled cubed sweet potatoes

2 tsp Worcestershire sauce, to taste

1 bay leaf

1 tsp ground thyme

1 tsp black pepper

500 gm chicken

1/2 bunch parsley (cut up and added at the end)

Spices to taste

ginger, chili powder, paprika, marjoram, and cayenne

Method

1 Combine all ingredients in a large pot.

2 Bring to boil.

3 Reduce heat to medium-low.

4 Cover and simmer for 25 minutes, until potatoes are tender.

5 Add chicken to soup mixture.

6 Add parsley

7 Remove bay leaf before serving.

8 Add spices to taste.

Note: If you prefer vegetarian soup, you can leave out the chicken and replace the chicken cube with a vegetable cube.

TRADITIONAL CHINESE MEDICINE AND WHAT IT SAYS ABOUT OSTEOPOROSIS:

Traditional Chinese Medicine (TCM) associates osteoporosis with the kidneys, the powerhouse (in TCM) for inborn Qi. In turn, inborn Qi is stored in the bones.

To treat osteoporosis, TCM doctors build kidney energy with acupuncture and herbal therapy. Qigong, an ancient Chinese energy practice, is an excellent way to develop your health because it helps the organs work more efficiently, and this helps your body save energy in the long run. It also recommends acupuncture to stimulate the kidney's energy. TCM also has ready-made herbs that are sold over the counter or on the internet that you might find helpful

TCM states that eating balanced and healthy meals also can improve your health. Food is an excellent resource, and it is relatively cheap. Many foods nourish the kidneys: **Walnuts, pine nuts, black beans, seafood—especially shellfish, and for osteoporosis, try making an old-fashioned bone soup. A recipe for an old-fashioned bone soup follows:**

VEAL JOINT SOUP

Veal Joint broth is excellent for calcium intake, osteoporosis, arthritis, and rheumatism. Veal joint broth supports the glands, stomach, ligaments, and digestive system and helps retain youth in the body.

Fresh uncut veal joint

3 onions

5 cloves

4 cloves garlic

2 sticks of cinnamon bark

5 cardamom seeds

3 star anise

3 stalks of celery, chopped

3 unpeeled potatoes, chopped

1 cup parsley, chopped

1 tsp cumin

1 tsp black pepper powder

Salt to taste

Method

In 1 tbsp vegetable oil, fry cinnamon, cloves, cardamom, star anise

Next, fry onions until they caramelize,

Add 1 liter of water and all ingredients (except salt), and ensure water covers all ingredients. You may pressure cook this for 30-40 minutes until it is soft.

If you do not have a pressure cooker, boil it until it becomes soft and comes off the bone.

When you think it is ready, add salt and more water to get the consistency you like.

STIR-FRY MUSTARD GREENS

2 teaspoons olive oil to stir fry

1 clove garlic

1 bunch mustard greens

2 tsp sesame oil

2 grape tomatoes (quartered)

1 tbsp vegetarian mushroom sauce

Method

Dice garlic and fry it lightly in a spoonful of olive oil.

Put a half cup of water in a saucepan and put the mustard leaves in to soften them.

Let the water evaporate.

Add the sesame oil and mushroom sauce.

Add the quartered tomatoes.

Note: You may do the same with any number of vegetables and greens that are calcium-rich.

Try this recipe with collard green, bok choy, swiss chard, watercress, or other greens.

CURRIED OKRA

1 onion

2 cloves garlic

1 tsp red chili powder

1 tsp turmeric powder

2 tsp lemon juice

7 okra - sliced about 1 inch thick

1 seeded red chilli (not the spicy variety)

Method

Fry the onion in 2 spoonfuls of vegetable oil, and add garlic (be careful not to burn the garlic).

Add chilli and turmeric powder and let it fry in oil well with the onions and garlic.

Add the okra.

Add the red chilli.

Remove from stove.

Pour lemon juice over okra and mix.

Eat with rice or whole wheat bread.

Note: Okra has about 50 mg of calcium per 100 grams. One onion has about 10 mg of calcium. Lemon has about 25 mg of calcium per lemon. So, just for this meal alone, you would get about 135 mg of your daily calcium if you eat it with a cup of rice (20 mg) or whole wheat bread (50 mg).

Do your maths, and you may be happy with the results. That is about one-fifth of your daily intake!

Note: You could also replace the okra in this recipe with leek. Both okra and leek have oxalic acid that interferes with calcium absorption, but this is minimal. Moreover, if you do not suffer from kidney stones, you are just fine.

LENTIL SOUP

1 1/2 cups lentils + 2 cloves garlic

3 cups water

1 onion

3 cloves garlic

1 tsp mustard seeds

1 tsp turmeric

1 red chilli, seeded

Salt to taste

Method

Boil lentils in 3 cups of water with 2 cloves garlic until they are soft and well cooked (add more water if necessary). Set aside.

Fry mustard seeds till they pop, add onions, and fry until fragrant; add 1 clove of garlic, turmeric, and red chili.

Add this fried mixture to a pot of lentils.

Bring lentils back to boil and add salt to taste.

Note: Lentils provide a good amount of calcium, about 100 mg, and onions are a great addition to the calcium treasure house.

There are many different kinds of lentils in the marketplace; you may try this recipe with any of these lentils.

TOFU IN COCONUT MILK

1 slab tofu – cut into 2cm cubes

2 cloves of garlic –crushed and minced

2 cm thick ginger sliced into strips (optional)

1 spring onion cut in 2cm lengths

I1 cup of coconut milk

2 cups of bean sprouts (green pea sprouts)

1 vegetable cube (dissolve in ¼ cup hot water)

1 red chilli sliced

Method

Fry the garlic in a spoonful of vegetable oil. Add ginger.

Add tofu cubes.

Put in vegetable cube that has already been dissolved in some hot water.

Add in bean sprouts, spring onions, and chili.

Add coconut milk and let it boil once before turning the stove off.

STIR-FRIED TOFU IN MUSHROOM SAUCE

1 slab tofu – cut into 2cm cubes

1 clove of garlic- sliced finely

2 cm thick ginger sliced into strips

1 spring onion cut in 2cm lengths

2 tbsp vegetarian oyster sauce or mushroom sauce

1 red chilli sliced (optional)

1½ tsp of sesame oil

Method

Fry the garlic in a spoonful of vegetable oil. Add ginger.

Add tofu cubes.

Add vegetarian oyster sauce or mushroom sauce and stir.

Add spring onions and chilli. Sprinkle sesame oil. Stir.
Serve hot

RICOTTA DIP

Ricotta is made with whey and is, therefore, full of calcium and all the other goodies that whey contains. This is a simple dip that is easy to enjoy. Mix the ingredients in all at once.

1 serving of ricotta

1 onion

1 grated apple

½ red pepper –minced finely

Salt to taste

Pinch of cayenne pepper

Dill –chopped

Method

Mix all the ingredients together.

Serve with chips or vegetable sticks.

A CONCOCTION TO MAKE PAIN IN THE BONES GO AWAY:

1 tsp turmeric

¼ teaspoon dry ginger

1 teaspoon fennel

1 teaspoon licorice powder

¼ teaspoon garlic paste

½ teaspoon fenugreek seed powder

Method

Mix and stir in a glass of water. Drink mixture 2 or 3 times a day. After 2 -3 months the pain in the bones will stop.

Note: This helps to balance the hormones and heals the pain in the bones caused by osteoporosis.

EGGSHELL CALCIUM RECIPE

Eggshell calcium has high bioavailability (the ability to be easily absorbed by the body). Synthetic calcium has low absorption rates, and so does dairy calcium, particularly if you are lactose intolerant.

Eggshells also have a high level of food safety. According to Dutch researchers, eggshells positively affect bone density when combined with other minerals such as vitamin D, Magnesium, and Zinc. There were measurable increases in bone density in the hip bones of the subjects after one year.

One eggshell makes about one teaspoon of powder and yields about 750-800mg of elemental calcium plus the other microelements, magnesium, boron, copper, iron, manganese, molybdenum, sulfur, silicon, zinc, etc. There are 27 elements in total. The composition of eggshells is very similar to that of our bones and teeth.

Method

1. Wash empty eggshells (make sure they are organic eggs!) in warm water until all the egg whites are removed. Do not remove the membrane.
2. Dry them thoroughly. Air-dry them for a few days in a clean place
3. Break them up into small pieces. Please put them in a dry grinder and grind them into fine powder.
4. Store the powdered eggshells in an airtight jar. Please keep them in a dry place.

½ a teaspoon = 400gm of elemental calcium. Put ½ teaspoon (½ tsp = 400gm of elemental calcium) in a dessertspoon and mix with warm water. Put it directly in your mouth and wash it down with water.

Note: Do not mix it in a glass of water because the eggshell powder is gritty and sinks to the bottom of the glass.

If you follow this booklet's advice, you will not need a magnesium supplement. If you are not, you may need approximately 400mg of magnesium.

Turning Eggshell Calcium to Calcium Citrate

The pure Eggshell form of calcium is calcium carbonate. If you want to turn it into calcium citrate, then here is what to do:

1. Take a teaspoon of the eggshell powder and place it on a small dish.
2. Mix it with the juice of ½ a lemon.
3. The solution will bubble and foam.
4. Leave it at room temperature for 6-12 hours.

It is ready to be taken. This is calcium citrate.

Calcium citrate is said to be more easily absorbed than calcium carbonate. If you think you need more food with magnesium, take a magnesium supplement of about 400.

What you have learned so far in Chapter 5: A recap

- The Key Recipe: to be taken every day
- The No1 Salad that you are to have daily: A Key Salad
- 16 recipes that should inspire you!
- A concoction to make the pain in the bones go away!

CHAPTER 6

PHYSICAL EXERCISE

The 5-minute powerful exercise that makes bones healthy!

Changing the diet alone is not enough. There has to be some physical exercise to compact those porous bones. But the trick is to have gentle exercises. If you are averse to exercising, then at least make time for 30-minute walks every other day. Also, try to do some stretching. A little yoga would do well.

The recommended exercises are weight-bearing exercises: your bones at this stage may be fragile, and you would have to be careful about such exercises if you are indeed stronger, then weight-bearing exercises are not an issue.

A SIMPLE QI GONG EXERCISE

I recommend a Qi Gong grounding exercise. It only lasts 5 minutes, but you must do it every day. Once you have the stamina, do it for 10-15 minutes.

This exercise in Qi gong is called The Horse: It is the physical act of balancing and stabilizing in a standing position. It also refers to the sensation of feeling safe and secure in the pose and the absence of instability or the sensation of being "off-balance." (which is what you are when you have osteoporosis; you are out of balance with the rest of yourself!).

This exercise borrows from the earth's energy to root yourself heavily to the ground. Here is how you do it:

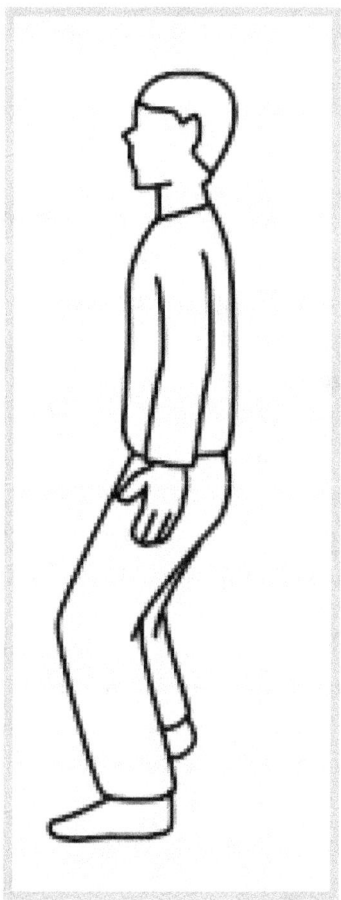

The Horse Stance

Breathe in

1. Stand with your feet shoulder-length apart
2. Bend your knees. At no time during this exercise
   must you lock your knees. Keens should be leaning
   out slightly.

3. The spine should be straight, the tailbone tucked in
4. All other parts of your body, particularly the thighs, back, and buttocks, should be relaxed
5. Visualise roots coming out of your free and going deep into the earth, anchoring you firmly to the ground. Feel balanced and stabilized, and the earth absorbs all negative energies
6. Without lifting your heels off the ground, start jumping up and down
7. Your arms must feel like the arms of a ragdoll, completely relaxed
8. After about one minute or so, when you are more comfortable with this exercise, you may lift your heel off the ground but not jump off the ground entirely!
9. Continue moving up and down in this manner, conscious of always relaxing your entire body. Do so for five minutes.
10. Most importantly, it would be best if you felt the looseness of your limbs.

You may initially be aware of the strain in your knee. If so, immediately relax. Eventually, your muscles will get used to this stance.

It is just moving up and down with your body in a particular position (in a relaxed manner) for five minutes.

This exercise will ensure that you are impacting your body such that the bones become stronger and you lose the porous section of your skeletal system.

You are in control of your life, your body, your mind, your soul, and your spirit.

Believe in your body's ability to heal itself. When you do, you are on your way to healing the "broken bits of bone" in your body. Make the skeleton strong again; there will be no more sponginess in your skeletal system, just solid and hard bones, just as nature made it to be.

Be determined to avoid foods that will negate the natural calcium you absorb. For example, avoid too much coffee (a cup a day is fine), carbonated drinks, and protein-laden foods like red meat. You can have them in moderation..., but do not go overboard.

Have the Key Salad every day and the Key Recipe with your breakfast every morning. Be inspired by the recipes that I have supplied you. Alternatively, be smart enough to eat foods rich in calcium, as listed in Chapter 4. Make sure you are eating enough sesame seeds. And if you think you need more magnesium, take a supplement. Not too much milk.

Exercise regularly. If you can, sign up for a slow yoga class that does not exert you too much. Just tell the yoga teacher of your condition first.

Promise yourself that you will do that five-minute exercise in Chapter Six.

Again, if you can sign up for a relaxed and easygoing Qi gong class, go for it!

Your feedback could be the encouragement someone needs to tackle overthinking and build resilience. By sharing your experience through a review on Amazon, you're contributing to a supportive community of growth and learning. Let's spread the positivity together! Here's the QR code for the book review page on Amazon. Just point your phone camera to it.

About the Author
Connect with me online at:

Twitter: http://twitter.com/amslucas
Naturalremediescentral@gmail.com

More books by AM Lucas
Foods that Heal Arthritis
Foods that Heal Inflammation